A PATH TO SUSTAINABLE LIFE SATISFACTION

◆◆◆

WORKBOOK

BY
DR. JENNIFER GUTTMAN

Published by Dr. Jennifer Guttman

ISBN: 978-0-578-20517-5

Book design: Kate Peterson // Pleasantly Progressive Design

TABLE OF CONTENTS

ACKNOWLEDGEMENT

As a lover of theater, I imagined that writing a workbook might be like drafting a script for a play. My vision was to follow my dream of utilizing the techniques that I've developed and refined as a psychologist to become a lifestyle coach/motivator. This project, "A Path to Sustainable Life Satisfaction," is part of a script that is still being written, which I finally found the courage to share with the rest of the world.

I firmly believe that achieving Sustainable Life Satisfaction is possible and I hope this workbook offers you the same guidance in your life that it did in helping me to complete it. I often tell people that I have never given a homework assignment that I didn't personally complete myself. So, as you go through these pages, you can rest assured that I tested and used every technique on my clients and myself. This provided great traction to demonstrate that I was onto something.

Like any great theater play, you have to have an amazing and supportive cast to help bring your vision to fruition, and I owe a lot to my incredible team. As with writing a play, initially there is the visionary. I met a guy in a restaurant three years ago and we began talking. He was instinctively passionate and believed in a mission for me that I didn't even realize could be harnessed. His inspiring encouragement helped give me the inner strength to take my first steps. He is my visionary and he knows who he is.

The cast grew and there are several other people who helped to guide me through the project development phase, drafting the text and walking me through the publication and distribution processes. Ramon Hervey II was the most integral of those people and I owe him a debt of gratitude too great to express here. The most I can do is acknowledge him for his support, patience and positive energy, and let you all know that he will always be the definition of a "closer" as I see it.

I want to thank Nicola Kraus for her collaborative talents and spirit through draft after draft, as well as being a great sounding board for many iterations of potential exercises. Kate Peterson's artistry and design helped to give the workbook the kind of professionalism and accessibility I hoped for. I want to thank James Weber for his beautiful photography and Christie Stone for her skillful styling. She is both a talented stylist and a true friend.

Throughout the writing process, I thought a lot about the woman who had mentored me. Dr. Eva Feindler provided both personal and professional guidance early in my career for which I will be forever grateful. I would not be the clinician I am today were it not for her. She taught me to live by the example you teach.

I've also been very fortunate to have people around me that I rely on to keep up the faith. I am grateful every day for my job and to have the pleasure to work with all my clients over the years who have contributed so much to my journey. They helped me develop Sustainable Life Satisfaction and have supported me through every step of this process. I am honored to have known each and every one of them. I talk about some of their stories in this workbook, but all of their stories have made a lasting imprint in my mind.

And lastly, there are my children, my true stars and the lights of my life. Steven and Alexa have been more supportive of every one of my endeavors then any mother has the right to hope for. I don't have the words to thank them appropriately, except to say that I would not be the person I am today without learning from and growing with them as their mother. Sustainable Life Satisfaction exists because of them. Alongside them, I have become more compassionate, curious, and patient. They continually help open my eyes to the commonalities and struggles we share and must endure to become our best selves. Their inspiration encourages me every single day. They are the joy in my most satisfying days.

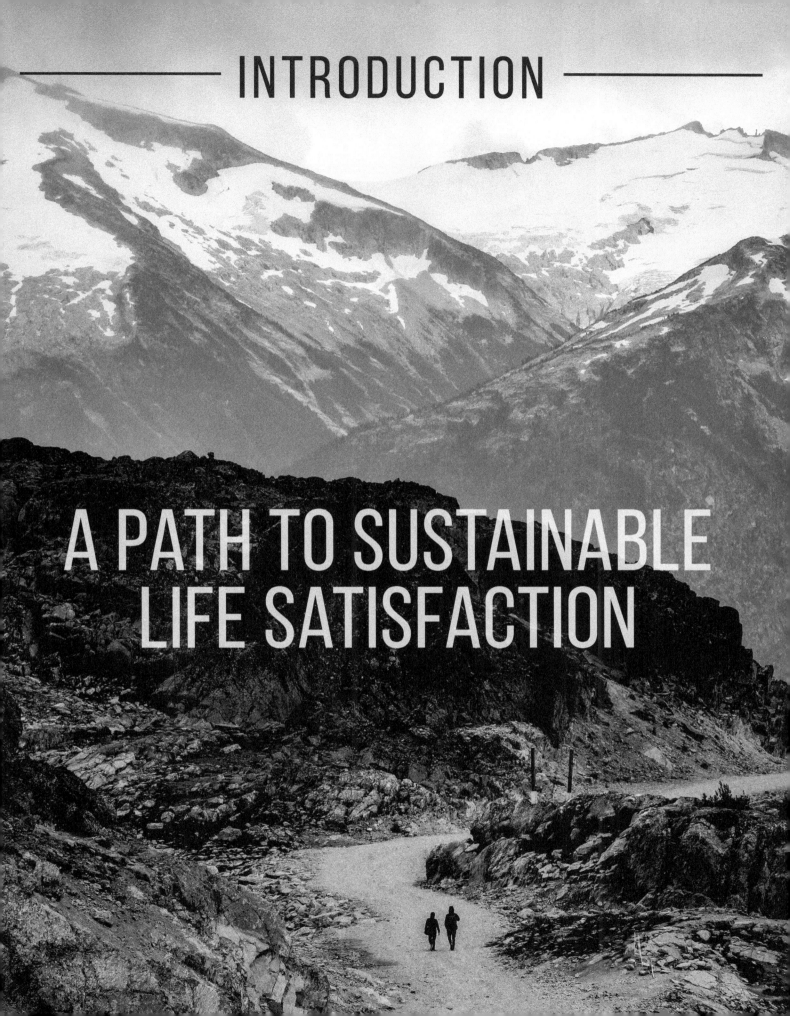

INTRODUCTION

A PATH TO SUSTAINABLE LIFE SATISFACTION

Todd was in his 40s when he came to me five years ago. Like many of the patients in my practice, on the surface it seemed like he had life figured out. Following his father's death, he had recently managed to sell the family business he had worked in for twenty years, was happily married, and had two healthy kids. So why had Todd's family given him the ultimatum of getting into therapy? Because now that Todd could finally totally self-direct his life, he couldn't get out of bed, his desk was in shambles, bills were piling up, and suddenly he couldn't "deal" with anything. He had achieved everything our culture tells us creates happiness, yet he wasn't happy. And worse, he was ashamed of not being happy.

As a Doctor of Psychology, I was seeing people like Todd every day in my therapy practice, people crippled by a core sense of inadequacy and self-loathing colliding against an impossible standard: happiness. "I should be happy." "I want to be happy." "I've read all the popular happiness books; why aren't I happy?"

So, I went the bookstore and bought the books my patients were reading. I followed the leading "happiness experts," trying to understand as much as I could about their approach, but something still felt off to me. I didn't see how to reconcile the happiness advice with my goal for my patients: a sustainable, unflappable belief in their inherent worthiness and lovability. And then I went back to my clinical foundation in Cognitive Behavioral Therapy and I looked at the scientific results my peers in this field were getting and something essential finally sunk in:

Our society is setting up people on a quest for failure because *happiness is the wrong goal.*

Happiness is a fleeting emotion, an endorphin rush, a chemical high. It's the moment the email comes in, the boss says yes, the first kiss, a picture on Instagram that only tells part of the story. It is *not* the foundation for a contented life. It does not equip you with the skills you need to navigate the endless challenges that everyone faces day-to-day. This is especially true in 2018, when the world seems more contentious, fractured, and just flat-out more frightening than ever before.

Then I looked at the clinically tested Cognitive Behavioral techniques and strategies I was teaching my patients and saw that they fell under six headings. They became the basis for my popular YouTube series, A Path to Sustainable Life Satisfaction. This workbook builds on those components: Starting Is Easy, Closing Is Hard, Decision-Making, Facing Fears, Reducing People-Pleasing Behaviors, Avoiding Assumptions, and Active Self-Reinforcement. In this workbook I want to start you on a journey to learn six simple exercises you can do today to begin incorporating these techniques and strategies into your life. They are behaviors that have had a profound impact on my patients' and my audience's quality of life and their ability to, not just cope, but thrive. That is the power of Sustainable Life Satisfaction^{SM}.

While sustainable happiness isn't a realistic goal, satisfaction can be achieved. In my practice, it became startlingly clear: these are the behavioral techniques that take my patients from being deeply unhappy, depressed, or anxious people who feel inherently unlovable, to being highly functional and deeply satisfied. The best part is that mastering them doesn't require in-person deep-dives with a therapist, they are practices anyone can do right now to change how they think, feel, and, ultimately, live. That is what I want for you in this workbook.

The exercises are designed to help build on what you may have learned from watching my web series and will take you through everything you would learn in private sessions with me at a fraction of the cost of even a single visit. The best part of Cognitive Behavioral Therapy is that it is action-oriented and exercise-based.

You can learn the six techniques just as well from me in a book as in a session. You can start applying the techniques right away. You can feel relief right away. And with consistent practice, you can achieve cognitive optimization, re-wiring your plastic brain to function in a new, more efficient and effective way.

In Chapter One I'll start by sharing the science behind why cognitive behavioral therapy is so clinically effective that it was the first kind of therapy ever to be covered by insurers. It is one of the best-studied forms of therapy and its benefits have been proven by trial after trial[1]. Once you understand that what I'm going to be teaching you has been scientifically proven to work, I move onto Thinking Errors and how to end them. From negative forecasting to an all-or-none paradigm, my patients have come to me making one or all of the most common Thinking Errors. By learning to take control of how your brain assembles information, you can actually start presenting yourself with a better outlook from which to work. Then I close out Chapter One by teaching you how to take back control of your emotions by modulating them using self-talk strategies. Thoughts create emotions. Emotions create distress. Relying on what we now know about neuro-plasticity, we can change how we think to create lasting changes in the brain. These techniques have given millions of people near-instant relief to their emotional distress and will revolutionize how you process the information coming at you every day, information we call life.

Then, chapter by chapter, I'll teach you my 6 Techniques of Sustainable Life Satisfaction: Starting is Easy, Closing is Hard, Making Decisions, Facing Fears, Avoiding Assumptions, Reducing People-Pleasing Behaviors, and Active Self-Reinforcement. By doing the exercises in every chapter, you will easily master the

---

[1]   *Robert Koch Institute (RKI). Psychotherapeutic healthcare. Berlin: RKI; 2008.*

techniques you can use in *any* situation to not only stay calm, but productive. SLS eliminates paralysis, indecision, and the self-loathing that underlies it. It enables people to tackle their lives proactively, and with every step forward they make, their sense of satisfaction grows. Their contentment grows. It becomes their bedrock.

After only a few months, Todd was able to break through his fear, make decisions, and close. He was not just getting out of bed and putting his affairs in order, but starting a new venture. In his home life, he was finally doing the things he had always talked about, taking his kids fishing and teaching them to play golf before the time with them got away from him completely. By learning how to actually follow his goals to completion he built up the self-confidence and self-collateral that let him know that he could handle starting a business without his father. He no longer needed that external approval to function.

Once my patients put these practices into action, they transform their lives; they switch careers, put themselves in the path of love, build community, and strengthen connection. But above all, they find a consistent contentment in their day-to-day lives, and a consistent belief in their inherent lovability that eluded them before.

Just don't call it happiness.

Like Todd and so many of my other clients, they're looking to increase their level happiness or to improve their self-satisfaction in various aspects of their lives. However, most people, whether they're in some form of therapy or not, are looking for the same things. The problem is they don't know how to self-evaluate to determine how much satisfaction they may already have in their lives. Now that you know a little bit about my brand concept, Sustainable Life Satisfaction, and the techniques I've designed to achieve it, I want you to take a simple Quiz before you read the rest of the workbook. The quiz, "Determining Your Level of Satisfaction In Your Life," is designed to help you make a realistic assessment of the level of satisfaction you have in your life right now. When you rate yourself, don't cheat, and try to be as honest with yourself as possible. Remember, the rating levels don't equate to being good or bad. It's a way for you to self-assess. As you go through each of the workbook exercises, you'll have a better understanding of how each of my techniques can benefit and help improve your level of satisfaction. Not happiness, satisfaction!

Store the Quiz in a safe place. After you've finished all the reading and doing all the exercises in the workbook, give yourself about a week, and then take the Quiz again. You can get a clean copy of the quiz by going to my website. Go back and review how you rated yourself, and see how your ratings' levels changed. In about a month, take the quiz again, and see if you're continuing to make progress in the areas that you feel are important to you.

ANSWER EACH QUESTION BY MAKING AN HONEST SELF-EVALUATION
BASED ON THESE FIVE (5) RATING MARKS.

1 — NEVER   2 — RARELY   3 — OCCASIONALLY   4 — OFFEN   5 — ALWAYS

_____ 1.   I can't make decisions on my own

_____ 2.   Often I feel like a fraud or an imposter at work

_____ 3.   I have problems finishing what I start

_____ 4.   I feel anxious a lot of the time

_____ 5.   I have trouble pushing myself to do things outside
              of my comfort zone

_____ 6.   I worry about what people think of me

_____ 7.   I'm easily frustrated or anxious when I can't predict outcomes

_____ 8.   I harbor resentment towards friends or family

_____ 9.   I have a tendency to put myself last

_____ 10.   I can't seem to figure out what I want

_____ 11.   I don't normally feel competent or worthy

_____ 12.   I struggle with being independent and self-reliant

_____ 13.   I'm unable to problem-solve for myself

_____ 14.   I find it difficult to cope with the unexpected

_____ 15.   I seek reinforcement from my supervisors and
              colleagues in the form of praise

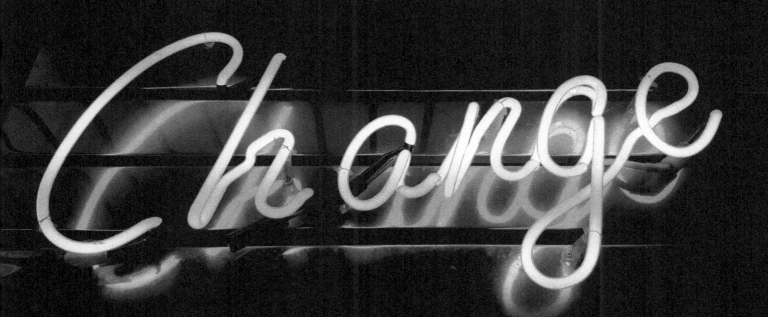

CHAPTER 1

HOW TO STOP THINKING ERRORS & ACHIEVE MOOD MODULATION

I'll never forget the moment I sat across from a patient and had an almost perverse thought, "She could be so happy, if only she wasn't so focused on … happiness." I was only one year into my private practice when I met Lisa. Lisa had been a very successful model in my youth, so her face was familiar. She was married to a British actor and they had four beautiful children. They lived on two continents and her children and husband were devoted to her. However, she was crushingly unhappy. She had tried multiple anti-depressant medications with no success and multiple outpatient mental health treatments, but continued to be plagued by feelings of inadequacy, insecurity, ineffectiveness, and fear. No amount of reassurance or love from the outside world could compete with her critical internal monologue. All she wanted was to be "happy" and couldn't figure out why an emotion that seemed like it should be so easy to grasp would be so impossibly out

---

OUR CULTURE'S CURRENT OBSESSION WITH "HAPPINESS" IS CAUSING SUFFERING.

---

of her reach. Over the years, this had sent her into an even greater sense of despair and self-disgust.

I believe that our culture's current obsession with "happiness" is causing suffering. You may also feel like you are trying hard to be happy—and failing. In an effort to reach that goal, perhaps you've read books on happiness, joined a meditation group, tried medication and/or diet modification. My patients arrive in my office having tried all of these and more. They have been working their butts off at "happiness"—and that's only making them feel worse. Because happiness is fleeting and, if that is the benchmark, the other 23 hours and 58 minutes of your day are going to seem pretty drab. What I have taught my hundreds of clients and thousands of online students is something much more practical, that can put your emotions, and, most importantly, your behavior back under your control.

So many of my patients want to be doing one thing but find themselves doing another. From big choices like career, to little choices like getting out of the office in time for family dinners, they have an intention, but life gets away from them and leaves them feeling...miserable. Then they go on social media and it seems like everyone they know has figured out the piece they're missing. They all have great jobs or the right partner, they all seem to be able to duck out in the middle of the day for the soccer game, they all seem to be doing it right. And now my patient is even more paralyzed with self-loathing.

And no amount of gratitude journaling is going to cut it.

After Lisa left my office, I looked at the range of what I was offering patients and where people were making the biggest strides, and realized all of the practical, actionable advice I was giving fell under one of six headings. There are the 6 principles you will master in this workbook: Becoming a Closer, Making Decisions, Breaking Through Fear, Avoiding Assumptions, Stopping the Need to Please, and Active Self-Reinforcement. I called this new goal Sustainable Life Satisfaction, or SLS, an action practice that can transform any life.

One of my patients adopted my 6 Techniques of Sustainable Life Satisfaction and made huge changes in how he lived and worked—and then his sister died unexpectedly. Happiness would have been a sabotaging goal under those circumstances, but he said to me, because he had been using my techniques, he handled the strain week in, week out, as best as humanly possible. He didn't hide in work, didn't numb himself with alcohol, food or TV. He made decisions for himself and his family, he saw each challenge through, avoided saying yes to things he couldn't actually take on, and didn't add drama to an already fraught situation by assuming the worst. And once he was through the immediate aftermath, he was proud of himself. He continued to do what all my patients do, build collateral with themselves that leads to core self-confidence and self-respect.

COGNITIVE BEHAVIORAL THERAPY IS THE MOST WELL-DOCUMENTED AND CLINICALLY-PROVEN THERAPY IN THE WORLD.

Starting in the next chapter, I'll be teaching you these techniques. But it's vital that you know before you begin that each one of these components is critical in achieving Sustainable Life Satisfaction; utilizing only one component will not give you the desired results you are searching for. Each works together and relies on the others to make dramatic cognitive shifts in the way you think, creating new neural pathways. Cherry picking some of them without others will not have the desired effect. It would be like strengthening one muscle but leaving the rest around it weak. You would actually leave yourself *more* prone to injury.

So, I trust that you will move through the workbook in order, learning all the techniques for maximum effect. Also, if you need additional pages, all of these exercises can be downloaded as PDFs off my website guttmanpsychology.com. But, before you can effectively incorporate them, I'd like you to know the science behind Cognitive Behavioral Therapy and why its been proven to work so well.

Cognitive Behavioral Therapy (CBT) is a problem-solving approach that modifies what we call "maladaptive" emotions, cognitions and behaviors. Meaning, if you find you are having emotions, thoughts, or behavioral responses to situations that some part of your brain is telling you aren't quite on the mark, CBT can help. Do you find yourself flooded with outsized emotions that seem excessive? Do you need to run worst-case scenarios all the time? Do you start a project when you're supposed to be getting out the door? These are all areas where CBT is extremely effective. CBT is the most-studied and well-documented therapy in the world[1] and has been clinically proven to work in countless studies.[2]

Self-Concept

One of the foundations of CBT is the very simple idea of the self-concept, originally introduced by Dr. Baumeister in 1998. How do we think about ourselves? What are our beliefs about ourselves and our attributes? These can have to do with gender, occupation, family values, family roles, or even hobbies. Most of my patients come to me with very low self-concepts.

The critical first step then becomes separating out, "This is how you think about yourself," from "This is who you *are*," because so frequently there is a

---

[1]   *Robert Koch Institute (RKI). Psychotherapeutic healthcare. Berlin: RKI; 2008.*
[2]   *Hoffman, The Efficacy of Cognitive Behavioral Therapy: A Review of Meta-analyses, Springer Science + Business Media, 2012*

disconnect. We have been thinking about ourselves or passing judgment on ourselves in one way for so long, we have stopped questioning the belief, or self-concept. This is the beginning of our exploration because once you realize that this concept is not who you *are*, but who you *decided* you are, you open the door to make a different decision.

Social Learning Theory

Developed in 1977 by Dr. Albert Bandura, President of the American Psychological Association, Social Learning Theory is based on the precept that people learn from each other via imitation, modeling and observation. I believe we learn the bulk of our behaviors from our parents. Parenting is a critical component in a child's development and in each chapter, I'm going to encourage you to consider, without judgment, what might have been modeled for you by your parents and ways in which that may have helped or hindered you. This is an important step because, once we start to look at our brains like a computer that was

WITHOUT A SENSE OF EFFECTIVENESS IN THE WORLD, HUMAN BEINGS CANNOT FIND SUSTAINABLE CONTENTMENT.

once programmed, we can choose to uninstall that program. It sounds simple, but it puts the power over your thoughts and behavior back in your hands.

Self-Efficacy & Self-Reinforcement

Bandura also discussed the importance of self-efficacy and self-reinforcement. Self-efficacy is an individual's belief in their capacity to execute behaviors. One of the greatest problems I see in my patients is they've lost the ability to believe that they can accomplish their goals. Then, gradually, they have let go of their goals altogether, leaving them feeling aimless and unproductive. Without a sense of effectiveness in the world, human beings cannot find sustainable contentment. The good news is that SLS develops and strengthens self-efficacy.

Self-reinforcement is essential because I strive to send my patients back out into the world knowing they only need themselves to stay successful in the long term. Through a cycle of execution and reinforcement they can continually strengthen their new practices until they're ingrained in their psyches and have become their new normal. You can do the same.

Co-Dependency

Co-dependency, as bestselling author Melody Beattie identified it, is when you find yourself dependent on reassurance and approval from others for your self-worth and identity definition. This dependence on an often chaotic outside world is not a recipe for sustainable contentment. Life is unpredictable. Our family, partners and community members are unpredictable. We cannot cede our power by needing validation or reassurance from them that we are living our best lives. I don't even like the saying, "A mother is only as happy as her unhappiest child."

That is giving a child too much power. It is much better to hold your ground as a content person, while making respectful space for their feelings and their journey. You want to stay in the boat, and pull others out of the water from there, not dive overboard after them.

Thinking Errors

There is no one on earth who does not engage in Thinking Errors. We all do it. After I explain the four major types, you will be amazed how often you will notice them coming up in everyday conversations. But, just because they're common, doesn't mean they're benign. In fact, in my clinical experience, Thinking Errors account for the majority of people's suffering.

What I'm going to be asking you to do here is akin to the film, *The Matrix*. My patients come to therapy with a strong conviction about how their lives are. They present to me a string of "facts," and the narrative of their lives

THINKING ERRORS DON'T EXIST IN A VACUUM.

THEY CREATE EMOTIONS.

that has led them to me.

And then I ask them to make a key shift.

Perhaps, those aren't the facts at all. Maybe, those are merely their *perception* of the facts. The ideas their brains created and clung to for self-protection.

As a species, we survived and evolved to rapidly make sense of every threat in our environment, to categorize every interaction and event, to assess and assign. We do it so naturally *we don't even notice we're doing it.* What leads to suffering is that we rarely stop to ask ourselves if what we've decided is wrong.

Because Thinking Errors don't exist in a vacuum, they create emotions. Thinking you're failing at something causes anxiety and despair. Thinking that an upcoming experience is going to be negative fills you with dread. These emotions live in our bodies. They come with increased heart rate, increased blood pressure, a constricted throat, crying, and/or sweating. These Thinking Errors end up leading us to *feel* awful.

There are four main types of Thinking Errors that I'm going to focus on here: Negative Forecasting, All-or-None Thinking, Magnification and Minimization. See which one feels like your default du jour.

Negative Forecasting

Negative forecasting is expecting bad things to happen. For example, expecting to go to a party and have a bad time; expecting to get a bad review; expecting that someone you haven't met yet won't like you. It can be seductive. We feel that if we keep our expectations low, we reduce the chances for disappointment. However, it is actually a toxic mental pattern because you are telling your brain what to look for and you are setting your outlook. Who wants to move forward into a future that is already pre-ordained to be bleak? It can cause depression and also alienate others socially, increasing isolation that becomes a self-fulfilling prophecy.

All or None Thinking

All or None thinking is looking at a situation in absolutes, with no grey areas. When a person does this, they use words in their head like "always" or "never," "best" or "worst," "perfect" or "failing."

I have a client, John, who came to me struggling to see any nuance in life. As he prepared to move to a new apartment he was stymied in decision making because he felt that the decisions he was going to make about what to order, what to pack, and when to have it delivered all represented critical choices that meant he was either, "being an adult the best and right way," or, "failing at it." The problem became that the pressure he was putting on himself to make these decisions with such absolutist rationale meant he didn't make any decisions at all. Avoidance became his foremost strategy. All or None Thinking can lead to a rabbit hole of indecision.

Magnification & Minimization

Magnification is making some small negative event very big in your mind. Let's say overall you received a 4 on your yearly review at work on a scale of 1-5, with 5 being the highest. However, one of the sub-ratings was a 2, which indicates "needs improvement." When a person is Magnifying, they only focus on the "2" rating and ignore the fact that the overall review "exceeded expectation."

Much has been written lately about our brain's negative bias, but to restate it here, the theory is that the humans who survived to pass along their genes focused on the negative. If you ate a berry that made you sick, forgot about it and ate it again, that second time might kill you. Whereas the person who ate the berry, got sick, and then avoided all berries, and warned their children about berries, lived to pass on his genes.

Magnification can feel comfortingly self-protective on some level. But it has consequences. Learning to shift focus away from these small slights can have huge behavioral impact, as we'll see in later chapters.

Minimization frequently works in tandem with Maximization, creating a negative feedback loop. Minimization is ignoring positive events. For example, someone is working at a new job and getting positive feedback for learning the telephone system, but he can only focus on the parts of the phone system that he still hasn't mastered perfectly, despite the positive feedback.

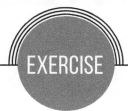
If you catch yourself with an elevated pulse, or a constricted chest, it's likely you are having a negative thought and I can almost guarantee that negative thought has an error in it. For that reason, it's critical that you do a forensic analysis of your thinking to identify and weed out your negative thoughts, and then balance the thought with a positive statement to counteract it.

The way you do that is as follows:

1. Identify the situation you're in:

     _____

     _____

2. Identify your mood:

     _____

     _____

3. Identify the intensity of your mood on a scale of 1-10 with 10 being the most intense your mood has ever been:

     _____

     _____

4. Identify your negative thought:

     _____

     _____

5. Identify the error type:

     _____

     _____

6. Balance the negative thought:

     _____

     _____

It's important to note that the error type is always related to the negative thought and *not* the situation. There are no errors in situations, only in the ways people think about situations. Just as a friend of mine from Alaska once said, "There's no such thing as bad weather, just bad clothes."

I know right now that might seem impossible. Clients say, "but what if my boyfriend breaks up with me?" That is an empirically sad situation. Although the mood rating may be high because of the severity of the event, that doesn't mean that you've necessarily escaped a Thinking Error, or two, that may be compounding an already obviously stressful situation.

Let's try two test cases so I can demonstrate what this looks like in action:

#1. Situation: I'm invited to a party Saturday night and I find myself suddenly wanting to have a glass of wine, get online, or check out in some way. What's really going on?

> Mood: I'm anxious.
>
> Mood Rating: 4. This isn't crippling, but it's uncomfortable.
>
> Negative Thought: "I won't have anyone to talk to at the party and I'm going to feel awkward."
>
> Error Type: Negative Forecasting
>
> Balance the Negative Thought: "When I go to parties I have more fun than I think I'm going to have," or, "I can find someone to talk to because I have in the past."

#2 Situation: I am going to have my performance review.

> Mood: Worried.

> Mood Rating: 3.

> Negative Thought: "I never get good reviews. My boss hates me."

> Error Type: All or None Thinking

> Balance the Negative Thought: "Is it true that I never get good reviews? Do I actually have any evidence that my boss has any feelings about me at all?" "No one expects me to be perfect except me." "No one can be perfect all of the time."

Thought Stopping

Another important Cognitive Behavioral strategy is Thought Stopping. The most famous thought-stopping technique uses a rubber band. The rubber band is placed on your wrist and when an errant thought arises, you snap the rubber band. Please don't snap so hard that you end up with welts on your arm, a slight sting is enough. This technique is meant to give mild punishment to your brain for engaging in a maladaptive behavior, in this case, a Thinking Error.

This may be hard to believe, but many of my clients say they snap the rubber band sometimes 500 times a day initially...telling themselves to "stop it" (meaning stop thinking the negative thought) and distract themselves. The fact is the brain does not like "punishment" and learns quickly, so 500 snaps a day quickly reduces as the brain accommodates by having fewer and fewer negative thoughts, for fear of getting the snap!

The benefit of a behavioral thought stopping technique is that you realize that you are in charge of your thoughts and not the other way around. You will come to recognize that you can encourage negative thoughts to continue or extinguish them. You have a choice to allow your anxiety to be in charge of you, or for you to be in charge of your anxiety. Once you realize that you are in charge, feelings of helplessness change to feelings of empowerment.

YOU HAVE A CHOICE TO ALLOW YOUR ANXIETY TO BE IN CHARGE OF YOU, OR FOR YOU TO BE IN CHARGE OF YOUR ANXIETY.

Mood Modulation

I cannot tell you how many of my new patients come to me overwhelmed or wrung out by their emotions. Their lives feel like a roller coaster of highs and lows, but predominantly lows. They are flooded with anger, sadness, jealousy, anxiety, and seemingly every occasion in their lives prompts this emotional tsunami.

My new client, Melissa, arrived one morning in my office, and she was beside herself. A mom she knew well had walked past her in the schoolyard without saying hello, her MetroCard suddenly wasn't working, and the barista had gotten her coffee order wrong. As she told me about her morning she was red-faced, her arms flailed, she spilled her incorrect coffee, and she was already strategizing about what to do about the "situation" with the other mom. One look at her and I could tell you her cortisol levels (our key stress hormone) were high and she was in fight-or-flight mode. It wasn't even 10am yet!

It took me a few weeks of working with Melissa to get her to see that how she felt could be brought under her control. In her mind, up until that point, things happened all day long that hijacked her mood. What I taught her was that she actually was making decisions at every turn about what was happening, and those decisions were creating her mood.

Negative emotions aren't harmless. They set off a chain of reactions inside our bodies that, over time, wear out our immune systems, lower our T-cell count[3], and leave us vulnerable to all sorts of diseases and syndromes. Also, when we are in that state we don't make decisions that diffuse problems, but rather exacerbate them. For example, by the time Melissa got off the train, she was so convinced she'd been slighted she sent that other mom a pretty harsh text. It turns out the other mom just had a lot on her mind because she was dealing with a sick parent. Now this other mom felt attacked and told other parents at the school. So, Melissa has gone from absolutely no situation at all to one of her own making. This was all because she picked thoughts that created emotions, in turn overwhelming her nervous system. Then, out of that discomfort she lashed out. You can see, this is not a recipe for Sustainable Life Satisfaction. So here I am going to teach you how to get your moods back under your control. It's vital for your overall sense of wellbeing.

---

[3] *Elenkov IJ (June 2004). "Glucocorticoids and the Th1/Th2 balance". Annals of the New York Academy of Sciences.* **1024** *(1): 138–46.*

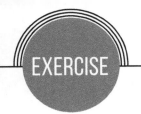

Just like hospitals rate pain on a 1-10 to effectively assess and treat it, you are going to learn to identify where, on a 10-point scale, your mood falls and how to appropriately match it to external events. Moods are rated on a scale of intensity and Events on a scale of severity.

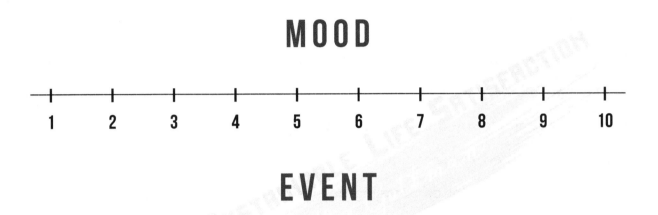

A 10 Event would be something like the death of a parent. A 9 would be your house burning to the ground. An 8 Event would be a full home burglary. A 7 would be getting fired. Daily arguments and issues with family members, peers, and co-workers fall between a 1 and 3 in terms of event severity. However, most of my patients come to me reacting to all events in their lives with an intensity level of something between an 8 and a 10. Now, how much credibility do you think a person has when they are reacting to daily stressors with the same emotional reactivity as they would to the death of a parent? Not much, right?

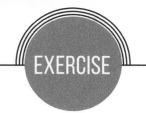
Poorly modulated mood states undermine our credibility, both to the outside world, and to ourselves. To the outside world, people that react too intensely to small negative events are considered dramatic or hysterical. More importantly, poor mood modulation undermines our internal belief in our resiliency in the world. It sets up a cognitive background where we believe we don't have the emotional landscape to cope with what we have to manage.

When you're in a situation and you can feel your mood escalating, ask yourself, "Over the course of my life does this level of an event warrant this intensity of a mood reaction?" If the answer is "no," then try to bring the intensity of your mood down to a level that matches the severity of the event. So, a level 3 event should garner a level 3 intensity mood rating and a level 1 event should garner a level 1 mood rating.

My clients do this by using a combination of self-talk around mood/event consistency, as well as identifying the Thinking Errors that are contributing to the poorly modulated mood. For example, what are the thoughts around a flight delay that are starting to make it feel cataclysmic? And can other thoughts be chosen?

Then they add one of the thought stopping techniques to stop the cycle of maladaptive thought patterns. By combining these techniques, you can learn to rein in your thinking and, by doing so, rein in your mood to match the level of the event.

Recovery Time

Measuring recovery time is a way you can determine how effective you are becoming at implementing this strategy. The shorter your recovery time from events that upset you, the better you're getting at being in charge of your thoughts and your mood.

For example, frequently when I first meet a client and I ask them how long it takes them to recover from an event that didn't go the way they had hoped, they will shyly admit that it took close to a day to recover. I ask them to start focusing on a goal recovery time of 20-minutes. If they want to win the Iron Man/Woman for recovery time they can aim for 10-minutes. It's amazing how people embrace challenging, but achievable goals!

Occasionally, I've even had calls from clients asking, "I just ended a relationship with my boyfriend, where do you think this falls on the mood-event consistency scale and how long do you think is

THE SHORTER YOUR RECOVERY TIME FROM EVENTS THAT UPSET YOU, THE BETTER YOU'RE GETTING AT BEING IN CHARGE OF YOUR THOUGHTS AND YOUR MOOD.

a reasonable recovery time to aim for?" This shows how much we have the ability to empower ourselves towards resilience, instead of despair.

If you can do this you will feel better modulated overall, gain a better perspective on what is really worth getting intensely upset about and, ultimately, feel better. *Sustainably* better.

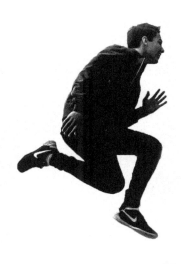

CHAPTER 2

STARTING IS EASY, CLOSING IS HARD

A PATH TO SUSTAINABLE LIFE SATISFACTION

Frequently, the first thing I notice about my clients is that they have trouble completing actions. They don't finish homework on time, don't study for tests, leave dishes in the sink, leave their apartments a mess, join the book club, but don't read the book, join the gym, but don't go, say they're going to switch jobs, apply to grad school, move, but never do. Then they look at the mess in their lives, or the health of their bodies, or their careers, and feel bad about themselves. By not closing they continually undermine their sense of self.

The truth is that starting tasks is easy, but closing is hard. This is because in the midst of every task, that adrenaline, that impetus to do the task wears off. Then you are just in the slog. The middle of the book, the 6am workouts, the moment where you have everything off your shelves, but haven't put anything away yet. That moment where you see that there is a lot of work between you and your goal.

Closing requires accountability, sustained effort, and organizational skills. However, learning how to accomplish those challenges is vital. The accomplishment comes with a sense of effectiveness and a feeling of self-efficacy, which develops into self-confidence, self-respect and a belief in your lovability. It's priceless!

BY NOT CLOSING, PEOPLE CONTINUALLY UNDERMINE THEIR SENSE OF SELF.

Why It's Hard for Some

As children and adolescents, we are reinforced by our parents for our creative ideas. This reinforcement is enough to make the actual *execution* of the idea seem unnecessary. Our parents also reward us for project progress. This support serves as enough reinforcement so that when the process becomes too boring, it's easy to abandon it.

As adults, the adrenaline rush we get from dreaming about a project feels great! We've all felt that experience of sitting around a table with friends scheming about the next billion-dollar idea, right? Mostly, the dreaming ends around that table, because acting on the fantasy is much harder than the table talk.

I had an art teacher once who was leading us on a museum tour. One of the students looked at a modern piece and said, "I could do that," and she shot back, "But you didn't. He did." What frequently separates the successful from the ambitious isn't talent, or quality of vision, but rather execution. This is why closing is such an important skill to master.

How to Set a Goal

Closing is obviously all about attaining your goal, but sometimes setting that goal is actually the problem. One of my clients, who was struggling in several areas of his life, had, for many years, wanted to buy an old car to tinker with the engine. He kept talking himself out of it because he wasn't sure if he could get it to work. So, I asked him, "Is it about tinkering or getting it to work?" What he remembered that he loved from childhood was getting under the engine with his dad, not driving per se. So, we decided that closing was simply getting the car to the driveway.

He bought the old car and the joy that working on it brought him flowed over to all the other areas of his life. Contrary to what his wife had feared, he actually became *more* involved with the family, and a better father. He became much more motivated at work and started making more money than he ever had before. And all that time, the car never left his driveway. Remember, it's not about how the world sees closing. YOU get to decide when the task will be done. One of my clients wanted to take an improv class, but her friends and family kept asking her what she was going to *do* with it? Finally, we decided that, for her, taking the class was the goal. The knowledge that she could decide, captain and execute this plan without worrying about others judging whether she utilized the skills she learned in the class, brought her a tremendous sense of fulfillment and personal effectiveness.

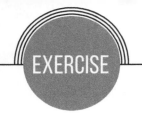
Write down in each category, everything that's not done that you wish was accomplished. You can also use scrap paper if you don't have enough space above. It could be one-off goals, like your wedding album, or routine behavior like cooking at home more often. Include all of it, so no self-deceit—this is not the time for cheating, but it's also not the space for judgment. However many items there are, there are. What's important is that you are taking this action here, now, to address them.

It can be a little overwhelming to see it all on a list, but also remind yourself this is it. It's all here now where you can look at it and tackle it. If you don't write it down, remember it will still be out there metaphorically taunting you anyway. Bills. Laundry. Wills. Health care proxies. Undonated outgrown clothes. Piles. Whatever your things are, write them down.

Then organize each list hierarchically one of two ways: by the length of time each item would take to complete or by the interest you have in completing each item. Also, you could arrange the Home list by time and the Social list by interest.

I then encourage my clients to do at least one thing they have avoided each day. Build momentum by tackling the items that either take the least time, or that you have the most interest in. It might just be taking out the garbage or watching a documentary you've been putting off. But see the goal all the way through to the end. And then cross it off.

Add to the list as needed.

Above all, don't set yourself up to fail. Make sure the time frame you're giving yourself is reasonable. It's better to have more time and complete less, than run out of time. If you feel like you're saying yes to doing something for someone

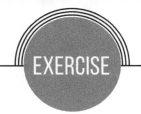
that you know you're not going to close, you've got to get comfortable with saying no. Not closing is too detrimental!

If there is something you keep putting off you may not really want to do it all. Let it go. One of my patients always thought she was going to be very involved with the PTSA, but by the time her children were in school full-time she had started a part-time business from home. She felt guilty, because she technically still had the time to volunteer, so she did, but, we identified, she didn't really have the bandwidth she thought she would. So, we empowered her to stop volunteering for things she was only getting done by the skin of her teeth or having to bow out of at the last minute. She felt she was disappointing herself on both fronts, not performing to her potential in her business, nor in her role on the PTSA. Once she gave herself permission to say no, she was more focused in her venture, made more money and donated more to the PTSA. Everyone was happy.

We all think we should be taking piano and learning Italian, but if that just doesn't really interest you deep down, let it go and find a goal that excites you. We all want to tell a parent or a spouse that we'll complete a chore for them, but if we're not going to follow through, say, "No." Help them find someone else to fulfill the task. Having an unattained goal hanging over your head for years undermines your sense of self.

Ultimately, effective closing is a stepping stone to developing a feeling of effectiveness in the world. It's about committing to keeping your life in order and honoring your word and what you'll find is that, as your self-reliance grows, so will your feelings of competence. Yes, it requires patience, yes it will change the way you think, but once you buy into it, your whole world starts to change.

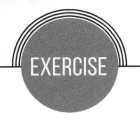

WORK

_____   _____

_____   _____

_____   _____

_____   _____

_____   _____

_____   _____

_____   _____

_____   _____

_____   _____

_____   _____

_____   _____

_____   _____

_____   _____

_____   _____

_____   _____

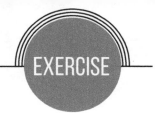

HOME

_____ _____
_____ _____
_____ _____
_____ _____
_____ _____
_____ _____
_____ _____
_____ _____
_____ _____
_____ _____
_____ _____
_____ _____
_____ _____
_____ _____
_____ _____
_____ _____

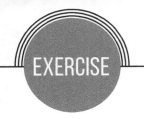

LEISURE

_____   _____
_____   _____
_____   _____
_____   _____
_____   _____
_____   _____
_____   _____
_____   _____
_____   _____
_____   _____
_____   _____
_____   _____
_____   _____
_____   _____
_____   _____
_____   _____

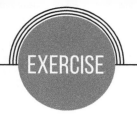
SOCIAL

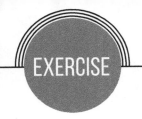

FAMILY

_____   _____
_____   _____
_____   _____
_____   _____
_____   _____
_____   _____
_____   _____
_____   _____
_____   _____
_____   _____
_____   _____
_____   _____
_____   _____
_____   _____
_____   _____

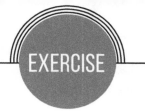

HEALTH

_____   _____

_____   _____

_____   _____

_____   _____

_____   _____

_____   _____

_____   _____

_____   _____

_____   _____

_____   _____

_____   _____

_____   _____

_____   _____

_____   _____

_____   _____

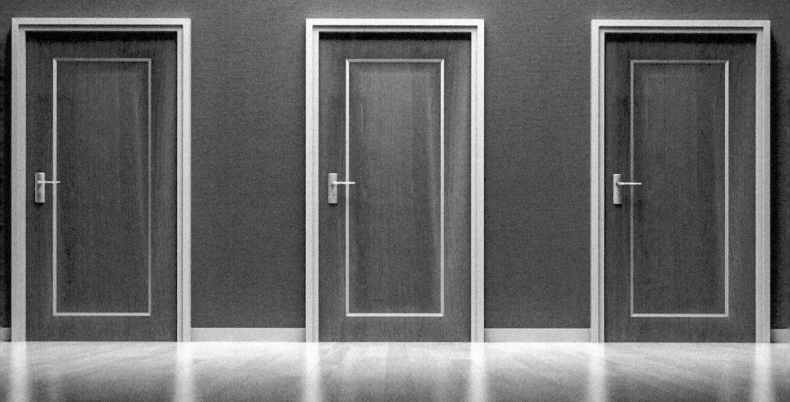

CHAPTER 3

DECISION MAKING

When I met Suri, a 20-something woman, her response to any question I posed was, "I don't know." She couldn't make any decisions. She couldn't decide which of two outfits to wear in the morning, or what to order in a restaurant. She consistently asked far too many questions at work, annoying co-workers and employers. Worst of all, she never had the courage to express an opinion about any topic, for fear of being wrong. Do any of you have a Suri in your life?

Many of my clients feel a profound sense of relief when they delegate decision-making to friends, like where to go to dinner or what movie to see or asking their parents to help make more important decisions, like what college to go to or what job to take.

Why is it so hard for some people to make decisions on their own?

Parenting in the Age of Terrorism

I see a sharp demarcation in my clients who were two or older on 9/11. Even for the very young among them, on an unconscious level, the world became a scary place. Parents felt like they could no longer predictably keep their children safe, and they started trying to mitigate that by being over-controlling. The instinct didn't come from a bad place, but it grossly undermined this generation's ability to function. Parents swooped in when life got challenging, and now these young adults don't know how to handle challenge. They haven't had to make many decisions, so they're terrified of making the wrong one. As the clinician, Madeline Levine, puts it in Teach Your Children Well: Parenting for Authentic Success:

> "While doing things for your child unnecessarily or prematurely can reduce motivation and increase dependency, it is the inability to maintain parental boundaries that most damages child development. When we do things for our children out of our own needs rather than theirs, it forces them to circumvent the most critical task of childhood: to develop a robust sense of self."

The problem is that when you don't get to make mistakes, and learn how to survive them, you don't learn to trust yourself. Across ages, across demographics, 85% of my clients struggle with basic decision-making.

In *Too Much of A Good Thing: How To Raise A Child Of Character In An Over-indulgent World*, Dan Kindlon writes:

> "Our children are lucky that they mean so much to us and that we have so much to give. [However], unless we raise them with the help of an inner parent who knows when to say no and be unyielding, our children will never develop the core strength, independence, and fortitude they will need to be happy. They will, in short, lack character; that unshakable sense of self that sees us through life's vicissitudes, and is the foundation of all our meaningful relationships."

We Are All Just Guessing

This is possibly the greatest illusion that I'm going to puncture in this workbook: no one actually ever makes a decision. We are always making a guess. It might be a very well-informed guess, it might be a guess we've made thousands of times, but today it might not play out the way it has before. Today the train might not have been faster. It might have been better to walk. Today that second cup of coffee might sour your stomach. Today the boss might have no patience with your sense of humor. Every day, minute to minute, moment by moment we are *trying* things. If you are someone who is afraid of making mistakes, it's so important to remember this. In today's glossy Facebook and Instagram world, everyone looks like they made all the right choices. *Oh look, they decided to travel with their children and look how much fun they're having!* When, in reality, their baby cried the whole plane ride and they actually bitterly regret their choice, but they're not going to post that. Everyone on social media looks like they have the perfect life. However, the operative words are "looks like." It's deceiving, it's propaganda, it's salesmanship, and it's meant to dupe you into believing that they have it all figured out. But, guess what? They don't. No one does. Everyone, and I mean everyone, is just guessing.

Now, going back to those parents who swooped in. It sets up a precedent in which the child, or even adolescent, really believes that the parent has all the answers. Newsflash: they don't. They're just guessing too! Maybe they're guessing with a little bit more life experience, but they're still guessing. They can suggest a college, but they don't actually "know" if it will be a good fit. They can suggest a career, but they have no concrete information that you'll love it. It's just a guess.

The problem with anyone guessing for you is that it's based on *their* life experience and *their* perspective. Their guess is filtered through everything that has ever happened to *them*. You're a different person, with a different set of dreams and aspirations. So, what worked well for them might not work as well for you.

EVERYONE ON SOCIAL MEDIA "LOOKS LIKE" THEY HAVE THE PERFECT LIFE. NO ONE DOES. EVERYONE, AND I MEAN EVERYONE, IS JUST GUESSING.

No Right or Wrong

There are no decisions in life that cannot be course corrected. It may be expensive, it may be time consuming, it may be emotional, but all decisions are reversible. Tattoos can be removed, careers, homes, colleges, and even marriages can be changed. You can always get off the ride. So, please, pick a ride because you won't know until you try.

One of my clients was paralyzed by the idea of having her long-term boyfriend move in. They had been together for years, but she didn't know if he was "the one." I told her, "There is no way around, but through." The only way to know was to try it, and if it didn't work out, New York is full of apartments.

Give yourself the freedom to know that it's better to cope with a mistaken choice and changed course, rather than never make a decision out of fear of the consequences. The consequences of giving into fear are much greater, which we'll learn all about in the next chapter.

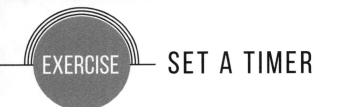
The second thing I teach clients is that laboring over a decision is a waste of precious mental energy. People should give themselves just enough time to gather information before making a decision. Of course, the time needed to do this is dependent on the decision being made. Some of my clients have been CEOs of companies, and when they've implemented this strategy, they are able to make major business decisions in under a few hours.

The strategy can also work just as effectively in making more mundane decisions. For example, if you go shopping for clothes, give yourself 10 minutes to choose what you're going to purchase. Decide what to order in a restaurant in 5 minutes. Gather information on what car to buy in 3 days. You get the idea? Second-guessing is not allowed, because there is no right or wrong answer.

Here is a list of self-talk phrases that I have found help my clients. Try them all and put a check mark next to the ones that help you.

_____   There are no right or wrong decisions.

_____   Decisions are reversible.

_____   I have the mental flexibility to change course.

_____   I have the ability to create alternatives if I don't like how it works out.

_____   Making decisions will make me more confident in myself.

_____   Everyone is just guessing.

_____   No one knows what's right for me better than me.

_____   I am the best person to decide the best course forward for me.

_____   Picking one path doesn't make the others disappear.

_____   Decisions aren't permanent.

If saying these phrases provokes anxiety, go to my website, www.guttmanpsychology.com and listen to my guided meditation to help relax and align your nervous system with this new belief. I have found that with consistent practice, most of my clients are able to change their decision-making habits within 3 weeks to 6 months. If it doesn't happen overnight, keep at it—change is coming.

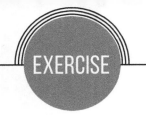
Think about an upcoming decision. What are the choices?

Write them down:

Option 1. _____

Option 2. _____

Is there a material difference between Options 1 and 2? If so what is it?

Write it down:

_____

_____

What does life look like if you make no decision?

Write it down:

_____

_____

Then I want you to choose one option, stick by your decision, breathe into any anxiety and trust your instincts. Try to ignore pressure from the outside world. Over time, evaluate how you feel about the decision. If you decide the decision worked out, great; if you decide it does not feel good, you have the power to do something different.

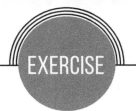
As you make decisions, write them down, so you build evidence and feel proud of your decision-making ability.

1. _____
2. _____
3. _____
4. _____
5. _____
6. _____
7. _____
8. _____
9. _____
10. _____
11. _____
12. _____
13. _____
14. _____
15. _____
16. _____
17. _____
18. _____
19. _____
20. _____

It may not be easy at first, but just start practicing by making a couple of decisions on your own every day. Start by making small decisions, like choosing a restaurant. Then move on to bigger decision-making, like not asking advice from someone about how to write a proposal at work or who to ask out on a date. You'll be surprised by how much more confident you will feel.

MAKING YOUR OWN DECISIONS LEADS YOU TO TRUST YOUR ABILITY TO COPE.

Remember my client, Suri? Well, she doesn't say "I don't know" anymore. We put a moratorium on that phrase early on, and now she has gained the confidence to make a lot of decisions on her own. She decides what exercise classes she wants to go to. If her friends join her, fine, and, if not, that's fine too. She decides what jobs to apply for and which night classes to take. She decides where she wants to eat when she goes out, or she decides what she wants to cook for dinner when she stays in.

Making your own decisions leads you to trust your ability to cope. The ability to cope will become pride, which will translate into feelings of self-worth and, eventually, a renewed belief in your lovability. Sustainable Life Satisfaction naturally flows from all of that.

CHAPTER 4

FACING FEARS

When my son was around 7 years old, baseball was "the" thing to be doing at recess, but he wasn't participating. This was causing him no small amount of stress. What I finally got out of him was that he was worried that if he swung at the ball and missed he would be embarrassed in front of his friends, so he was too anxious to try.

At first, I tried telling him what I had always told myself, "Steven, face your fears." But he came home and said that watching the kids play baseball and not participating *was* like looking fear in the face and it didn't feel good at all.

So, then I said to him, "Steven, what about finding out what's on the *other side* of your fear?" He didn't totally trust me, but he was willing to give it a shot because anything was better than how he felt at recess. The next day, heart pounding, he pushed himself to take a turn at bat, telling himself that, whatever happened next, at least he would be on

FROM THAT
DAY FORWARD,
THERE WAS NO
STOPPING HIM.

the *other side*. He actually did hit the ball, but, he emphasized to me that night, that wasn't the important part. "The important part is that the other side of fear feels GREAT!!!" To get that feeling, you are going to have to walk through your fear.

From that day forward, there was no stopping him. He ran around challenging himself to greater and greater tasks that induced anxiety and fear to show himself that he was capable of coping with anything. It's amazing, now that he's 18, how he initiates conversations with authority figures and is not afraid to advocate on his own behalf. And this is not about arrogance or hubris; he's actually quite humble. What this is about is his ability to compartmentalize his ability from his fear. He doesn't allow his fear to hinder his progress in tasks that are naturally anxiety provoking, instead he uses the energy from that fear to propel him forward in a positive way. It sounds like an oxymoron, but mastering discomfort is the doorway to a lifetime of satisfaction. In that way, his fear is his sous chef.

Why Many Adults Let Fear Stop Them

Once again, like indecision, this frequently has its roots in childhood programming. Parents don't like to see their children anxious or distressed. For this reason, when a child or adolescent looks uncomfortable in a given situation, it's not uncommon for a parent to swoop in and rescue their child from the situation. However, it also doesn't show the child or adolescent that they are capable and competent and that they can survive feelings of insecurity and overcome them. Although this is done with the best of intentions, what it's actually reinforcing is the need to be rescued.

Now it's time to learn that you can rescue yourself in fear-inducing situations because you have the coping skills to do it.

Coping

Coping is your belief that, in any given situation, you can figure out where the exit door is. The vast majority of my patients come to me with the belief that they walk into rooms without exits. But I am here to tell you, every room has an exit. It can be hard to find sometimes, especially if the room looks different than you expected, but there is one.

The only way to find it, however, is to stay calm. Otherwise your animal brain takes over, your limbic system is engaged, and you are back in fight-or-flight mode. Remember Melissa? You never want to take action from that triggered state.

Instead, remain calm, identify the problem, and then look around for the creative solution. If you believe you have the capacity to do so, you *will* find the solution. This is why it's vital, if you don't have that belief, to start practices that will cultivate it within yourself. It may not be the exact same solution as you initially started out with, but the new solution you discover will likely be close enough to suffice.

Let's talk about John again for a second. Do you remember him from Chapter One, the section on All or None thinking? I asked him, what would happen in his black and white world if the bed was not delivered on time, despite his best intentions.

He looked perplexed and said, "it will be because I made sure." I explained to him that unfortunately the world often doesn't work as smoothly as we hope. Assuming the bed will be delivered just because it's supposed to be, doesn't allow John to consider the possibility that it might not be. Thus, he is not prepared to cope if there's a problem. In that way, he diminishes his belief in his coping ability by so firmly believing in his control of the outside world. I asked him if he thought he could figure out an alternative solution should the bed not come on time. In the relaxed setting of my office, of course he could.

Then I proposed a hypothetical situation. The bed is not delivered on time and you have to implement that alternative solution. A week later, are you going to harp on the fact that it was delivered late, or are you going to be proud of yourself for taking care of it. Without missing a beat, he said, "I'd feel proud of myself for handling the situation." This demonstrates the personal power found in coping rather than control.

Subjective Units of Distress

Have you ever been to the hospital or doctor and they ask you to rate your pain on a scale of 1-10? We have a similar scale that we use in Cognitive Behavioral Therapy, but it's called Subjective Units of Distress, or SUD, and it measures emotional pain on a scale of 1 to 100. Similar to the Mood Modulation Scale from Chapter One, many people rate all their emotions near the 100-level mark, but our goal in the next few exercises is to bring your fear levels down to as close to the 0 mark as possible.

List the Top 20 things you avoid out of fear and their SUD level:

1. _____

2. _____

3. _____

4. _____

5. _____

6. _____

7. _____

8. _____

9. _____

10. _____

11. _____

12. _____

13. _____

14. _____

15. _____

16. _____

17. _____

18. _____

19. _____

20. _____

Now that you are looking at them out here in the open, we can start to tackle them, one by one, so you don't have to waste any more energy avoiding people or activities who truly have no power over you.

DE-ESCALATING STATEMENTS FOR FACING FEARS

Self-talk can be hugely helpful for facing fears. When you find yourself wanting to avoid an action out of fear, try repeating one of these statements until you feel capable:

1. I'm in charge of my fear, it's not in charge of me.

2. Fear is my co-captain.

3. Fear is my sous-chef.

4. Conquering fear makes me feel powerful.

5. The more I challenge myself to face my fear the more confident I feel.

6. I'm not going to diminish my belief in myself anymore by avoiding things.

7. I'm stronger and more powerful than I think.

8. I'm going to channel the energy I get from fear into positive action.

9. Fear does not equal danger; it's more about me than the situation.

Making Fear Your Sous-Chef

I start every morning by asking, "What fear am I going to face today?" When I started doing this I would drive places without the GPS, relying solely on my own intuitive navigation system, I'd start conversations with strangers, and, one time, I managed to slide down a particularly daunting waterslide in an amusement park! I suggest starting with simple fears, like making a telephone call you've been avoiding, going somewhere new or simply saying, "Yes," to an activity you would normally avoid.

Try to lie in bed for that extra minute before getting up and mentally scroll through your day to identify where you may be able to face a fear and then "close." You will be amazed over time at how much more confident you will feel.

FACING A FEAR EVERY DAY IS IMPORTANT BECAUSE IT WILL MAKE ATTAINING ALL YOUR OTHER GOALS THAT MUCH EASIER.

Facing a fear every day is important because it will make all your other goals, closing, decision-making, and saying no, that much easier. It should become part of your routine, like brushing your teeth. The more habitual it becomes, the more you will feel like you can conquer any challenge that life puts in front of you.

As your ability to face challenges grows, so will your belief that you have core strength, which leads to an inherent sense of value. This value is also what I call lovability, the unshakable faith that we are worthy of love and belonging.

	FEAR	SUD LEVEL 1-100	HOW YOU TACKLED IT	SUD LEVEL AFTERWARD 1-100
MONDAY				
TUESDAY				
WEDNESDAY				
THURSDAY				
FRIDAY				
SATURDAY				
SUNDAY				

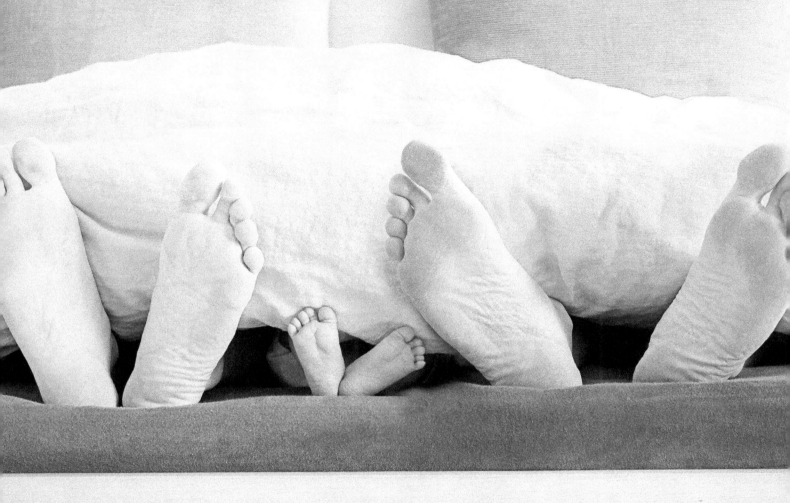

CHAPTER 5

AVOIDING ASSUMPTIONS

Many Cognitive Behaviorists call the process of avoiding assumptions, negative forecasting, which we covered in Chapter One. In my view, negative forecasting means that you expect bad things to happen. Assumptions are different in a critical way and learning not to make them can unlock powerful change in your day-to-day life.

What are assumptions? They are guesses, or predictions, based on a little bit of information. The problem with assumptions is that, far too often, they are wrong. When you take action based on erroneous information, you are setting yourself up for a toxic situation. Think back to Melissa and her feud with a fellow mom based on the assumption that she was being snubbed. If she had reached out to get information before she acted, she could have avoided bringing more drama and stress into her life.

OUR SURVIVAL RESTED ON OUR PREPAREDNESS, ON OUR ABILITY TO MAKE ASSUMPTIONS.

BUT NOW IT UNDERMINES US MORE THAN IT SERVES US.

When Assumptions Served Us

For thousands of years, as our brains evolved and developed, our survival centered around the cycle of the sun and how that impacted our food sources. We evolved to predict, to plan to do next year what worked this year. Most of the time it served us. All over the world, we developed planting and harvesting seasons. We figured out how to read nature to predict storms, hot seasons, cold seasons. Our survival rested on our preparedness, on our ability to make assumptions.

But now it undermines us more than it serves us.

In reality, people are not just one of four seasons. They are easy to misread.

As children, we desperately want to make our parents proud of us. We start guessing about what they might think about us and gauge our behavior based on our guesswork. When they give us positive feedback, we value our ability to make assumptions. Then, armed with our own sense of how good we think we are at this very maladaptive behavior, we go out into the world. We attempt to utilize this behavior in many interpersonal relationships to reduce the potential for emotional pain.

But when you come into a situation with a lot of what people commonly call "baggage," you are reading the situation based on your own history. A history the person across from you may have had zero role in shaping.

For example, I cannot tell you how many of my clients go into dating situations with negative assumptions about their date's behavior because of past experience. "He said he was running late because the train was delayed, but I've been here before; he probably just didn't care about holding me up. He was really apologetic when he arrived, but I was cold to show him I didn't appreciate it." Now, if he really was stuck on a crowded train, her negative assumptions have just sunk the date before it started. This is all because of her history with other people's behavior, for which he is not responsible.

The Chess Game

I cannot tell you how many people sit across from me every week and say something similar to this story from my patient, Stacy: "I want to host Sunday dinners with my family, but there is no way my mother-in-law is going to go for that. What I'm going to do is refuse to go to my mother-in-law's, forcing my husband to choose between the two of us. He's going to choose her and I'm going to be left behind while her takes our kids to her house."

Do you see the chain of assumptions? She was so many moves ahead, effectively bringing herself to the brink of a family war—all in her mind.

Once I encouraged Stacy to take the first step *without* any assumptions, guess what happened? Her mother-in-law was actually tired of hosting Sunday dinners; it had become too much work. She was happy to come into the city and see them for brunch instead.

The reason it's so important to go into situations, especially conflicts, without assumptions, is that, with assumptions in place, people go into the first round full of either hostility, defensiveness or sadness. They are assuming that their needs won't be met.

More often than not, this is a self-fulfilling prophecy.

Trust Your Ability to Cope

We act on assumptions because we don't trust in our own ability to cope with whatever the other person may be thinking or whatever action they may take. For this reason, we engage in preemptive coping, as if this will better prepare us should the imagined situation ever arise. This is because of our inherent feelings of inadequacy and ineffectiveness in the world.

Once you stop acting based on assumptions, you'll force yourself to cope with the fear and insecurity. You'll also have to learn to wait for a situation to unfold organically. If you can do that, your feelings of competence will improve. You will also realize you have the ability to effectively handle situations without anticipating future outcomes. Once you eliminate working so hard to figure out whether people's actions or thoughts are working against you, you'll naturally feel more content. Just remember you only have control over yourself. You can't control other people's thoughts, feelings or actions.

JUST REMEMBER YOU ONLY HAVE CONTROL OF YOURSELF.

Learn to Sit with Not Knowing

The other factor that drives our love of assumptions is our inability to sit with uncomfortable feelings, and no feeling is more uncomfortable than not knowing where you stand or what the outcome will be. People tend to rush to bad outcomes, rather than wait for real evidence to come their way. In one of my favorite movies, *Tootsie*, Terri Garr, who is in love with Dustin Hoffman, says to him,

---

LEARN TO CULTIVATE PATIENCE.

"There is rejection in every relationship. I would just like my rejection now." We would rather push for our worst-case scenario to come to fruition than sit, expecting it. So, the key is to sit without that expectation.

Learn to cultivate patience. Patience is a trait very few of us don't need to work on. Wait for the evidence and don't act until you have it. If the evidence never comes, you do nothing. This will feel very uncomfortable at first. When you feel anxious, remember that you have absolutely no idea what's coming next. Breathe into the unknown.

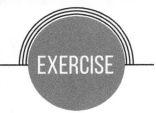

The first thing you need to do when you've made an assumption about someone else's behavior or intentions is: "find the evidence." And by evidence I truly mean something admissible in a court of law. Not a facial expression, not body language, not a feeling. Actions and words. Unless there is physical or verbal evidence of a thought or action from another person, you'll be operating based on a projection of your own insecurities. We also do this because we don't like the fear we experience from not knowing what another person is thinking or what they may do.

On the next page, write down any assumptions you have, and then ask yourself if there is hard evidence to back up that assumption. If the answer is no, I want you to pick one of the Thought Stopping Techniques from Chapter One and do it until your thinking is once again supported by concrete evidence.

When you're not worried about what other people are thinking about you, you'll be better able to focus on how you feel about yourself. As your insecurities fall away, they'll be replaced by feelings of self-confidence and lovability. This will lead to consistently greater feelings of life satisfaction than you could have ever imagined.

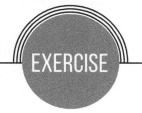

ASSUMPTION LOG

ASSUMPTION	EVIDENCE (YES/NO)	THOUGHT STOPPING TECHNIQUE

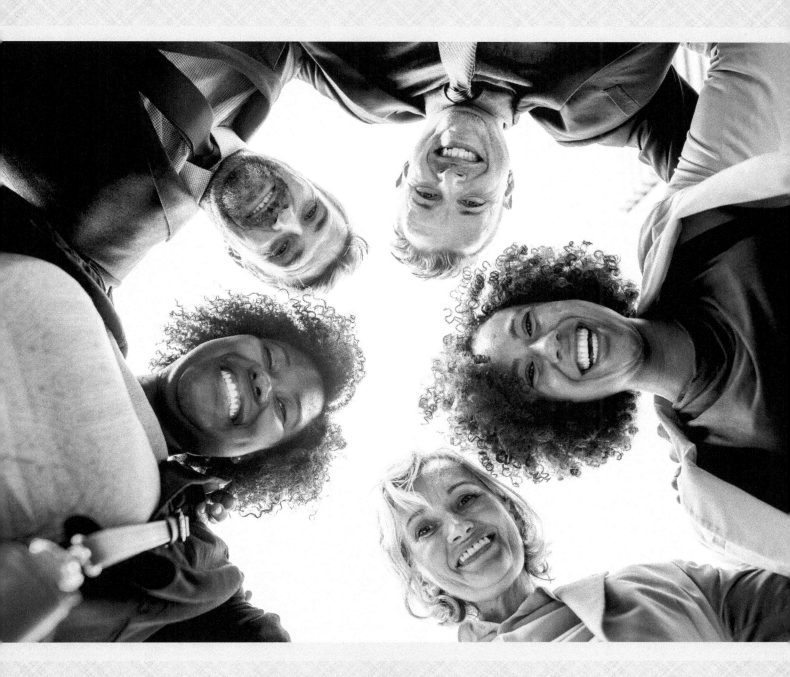

CHAPTER 6

REDUCING PEOPLE-PLEASING BEHAVIORS

The woman who inspired me to study the importance of people-pleasing behaviors on human interaction is not a psychologist. She is an integral member of the recovery community and well known for her books on co-dependency. Her name is Melody Beattie. As I studied and learned about co-dependency, I realized that utilizing that term to apply only to the recovery community seemed too narrow. Most of the behaviors that she identifies as indicators of co-dependency are typical of all of us.

PEOPLE-PLEASING CAN TAKE MANY FORMS.

So I started asking my clients to review Beattie's list of co-dependent behaviors and identify which ones applied to them. Circle the ones that apply to you. They include:

1. Difficulty being alone

2. Feeling responsible for other people

3. Feeling compelled to solve other people's problems

4. Over-anticipating other people's needs

5. Saying, "yes" when you mean "no"

6. Not knowing what you want or need

7. Doing things for others that they are capable of doing for themselves

8. Feeling that you spend your whole life giving without reciprocity

9. Feeling attracted to needy people

10. Feeling victimized and under-appreciated

11. Having difficulty making decisions

12. Feeling a lot of guilt and shame

13. Feeling unlovable

14. Having an overwhelming desire for acceptance and affection

Almost everyone comes to me exhibiting some of these behaviors. But in this chapter, I want to focus on just one co-dependent behavior, people-pleasing.

People-pleasing can take many forms. One form is anticipating others' needs and putting those needs above your own. A second, and much more subtle form, is imposing your help on others. We all know someone like that, someone who has gotten their sense of self-worth their entire life from over-extending themselves to the point that they can no longer tell if their help is even wanted. They are compelled to jump in and start "helping," even to the detriment of their own wellbeing and the wishes of their recipient. And then they get angry when their action isn't reciprocated or appreciated to the extent they think it deserves to be.

Many of my patients have co-dependent parents from the Baby Boomer generation. Women who were raised to put everyone's needs ahead of their own, but now direct a lot of rage at their adult children because their need for accolades is bottomless. My patients feel endlessly confused. "I don't understand, I didn't ask my mother to come to my apartment and do my laundry and now she's so angry at me!" That is co-dependence.

The Origins of The Need to Please

Beattie notes that this behavior starts when we're children. Sometimes in families the implicit or explicit message is to put others before yourself. It could have been a way to manage a volatile home life, step in for parents who weren't fully mature themselves, or make an out-of-control situation feel manageable. Think of the child who starts preparing dinner at a young age because the parents can't—or won't. This child grows up to over-extend themselves in every way to create order.

Managing volatility can be self-reinforcing because it creates a sense of purpose, value and self-worth in a maladaptive way. For this reason, a child may go on to use this behavior in future relationships, believing that it will secure a sense of indispensability, arresting fears of abandonment. But this is an unsustainable coping mechanism that will ultimately be counterproductive.

How to Stop

To stop, you must learn to look inside yourself for the reinforcement and reassurance about your worth that you've been seeking from others. Beattie notes that the most comfortable people to be around "are those who are considerate of others, but who ultimately please themselves."

I recommend this formula to my clients: first, try to stop guiding, problem-solving, making suggestions, offering advice or doing things for your family and friends unless you're *specifically* asked, as in, "Jennifer, will you do X for me?" or "Jennifer, what do you think I

> DON'T DO ANYTHING THAT YOU DON'T WANT TO DO, SIMPLY BECAUSE YOU'RE HOPING THAT YOU WILL GET THE SAME TREATMENT DOWN THE LINE.

should do about X?" Otherwise, just listen.

This is going to be very difficult if you're used to making yourself feel comfortable by launching in with "help" in the form of offering advice or running errands. But it's ok to be compassionate without offering unsolicited advice. Remember, the reason you want to stop this behavior is because it sets you up to want/need gratitude or reciprocation, which can lead to potential disappointment and resentment.

Next, don't do anything that you don't want to do, hoping that you will get the same treatment down the line. Remember, people cannot be relied on to treat you the same way that you treat them. That expectation is unreasonable. You also should not do something for someone with the hope of being appreciated or receiving accolades from others for your behavior, because reinforcement from the outside world is not reliable.

Lastly, do things you want to do for family and friends because you want to do them. Do them because you have the time and it doesn't interfere with anything else you have planned. Do them knowing that it's unlikely you will receive anything in return immediately or in the future.

Praise Yourself

The next step is to learn how to please yourself. When you're not getting the reinforcement you need from others, remind yourself that you're a good friend, daughter, son, or partner. Remind yourself that you're compassionate and kind. Don't look to others for positive feedback. You are the only one that needs to believe in you. If you don't, no matter how many times others tell you, the message will never translate to a belief in your lovability or life satisfaction. If the focus of control is on the "other" for reinforcement of your value, then any feelings of life satisfaction you have will always be transient.

I have a client, Amy, who came to me struggling mightily with this concept. Amy regularly delegated reassurance of her self-worth and value to family and

---

YOU ARE THE ONLY ONE THAT NEEDS TO BELIEVE IN YOU.

---

friends. She demanded a lot from them: praise, assistance, and even gifts. If what she demanded wasn't forthcoming, she fell into regular states of despair. She felt she was a generous giver to others and couldn't understand why she never felt adequately or effectively filled up, or taken care of by other people. No matter how much direction she gave them about how they could effectively demonstrate their love to her, their efforts would always fall short in some way. She was perpetually resentful and disappointed.

On the surface, one could have looked at her with a critical eye as needy and high-maintenance; however, if you looked deeper, Amy was a woman who was extraordinarily insecure, wracked by feelings of inadequacy and low self-worth. She was running around trying to do for others in a desperate attempt to justify her value, harboring an unrealistic hope that their failed attempts to show their appreciation would fill her bottomless well of self-criticism and doubt.

It's been a slow process for her, but Amy's been working diligently to re-train her brain to focus on her own actions, such as continuing education classes. This helps her develop pride in personal accomplishments, instead of using others' appreciation or presents as a barometer for her merit.

Learn to Love Your Own Company

Not fearing loneliness is a great way to reduce people-pleasing behaviors. Practice going to a movie or out to eat alone. I know it seems hard, but it's not as hard as you think. Shop alone and pick out something you like without asking anyone's opinion. Most importantly, don't break plans you make with yourself. It sends a message that a plan you make with yourself doesn't hold as much value as a plan you make with someone else. This backhandedly decreases your value.

BELIEVING IN YOUR INHERENT LOVABILITY MEANS KNOWING PEOPLE WILL STILL BE THERE FOR YOU EVEN IF YOU HAVE NOT MADE YOURSELF INDISPENSABLE TO THEM.

If you plan to go running, don't cancel on yourself...go. If you plan to go to a movie, don't cancel on yourself...go.

You must value your own company and trust that people will not abandon you, even if you don't drop everything for them. Believing in your inherent lovability means knowing people will still be there for you even if you have not made yourself indispensable to them, or frantically searched for ways to please them. Adding this to the tools I have already taught you puts you farther down the road to achieve Sustainable Life Satisfaction.

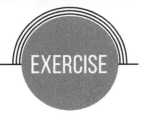 EXERCISE — PEOPLE-PLEASING CHECKLIST

How much does this chapter apply to you? Answer the questions yes/no and then tally your number of yes's.

DO YOU FEEL…	YES/NO
1. Like you never have privacy?	
2. Like you're never listened to?	
3. Like you're overly sensitive?	
4. Like you don't have control?	
5. Like you put your needs last?	
6. Unfairly criticized?	
7. Resentful?	
8. Fear of being replaced?	
9. Lonely?	
10. Insecure?	
11. Taken for granted?	
12. Bored when alone?	
13. Over-committed?	
14. Under appreciated?	
15. Anxious?	

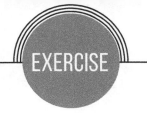
IF YOU SCORED BETWEEN 1-5

"At Risk." Nurture your sense of self-worth. Attend to the exercises in this chapter.

IF YOU SCORED BETWEEN 6 AND 10

"Danger Zone." You may already be in the process of losing your sense of self as you subserve your needs to others. Prioritize the exercises in this chapter as you proceed down the Path to Sustainable Life Satisfaction.

IF YOU SCORED BETWEEN 11 AND 15

"Enmeshed." You probably have already developed a habit of suppressing your needs while elevating the needs of others. This process may be occurring so quickly, it feels almost unconscious. It will take patience to change these habits as well as an ability to tolerate the fear that comes with separating your identity into an autonomous self. You can do this, but it will take time and small steps. Praise yourself for progress and try not to be put off by how exhausting and challenging the task may be at times. The closer you get to independence, you will realize that your effort is going to pay off in more ways then you ever imagined.

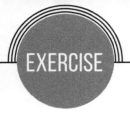
How often do you feel resentful? (Circle one.)

    Most of the time

    2-3 times a week

    At least once a week

    Rarely

Describe the situations that make you resentful:

_____

_____

_____

Describe the people you feel most resentful around:

_____

_____

_____

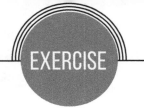
Mark which ones you're doing now. Ask yourself:

	YES/NO
Am I offering unsolicited advice?	
Am I changing my plans to accommodate other people?	
Am I resentful because people don't treat me the way I treat them?	
Do I feel like I always come last or suffer "invisibility syndrome"?	
Do I make time for myself?	
Do I mindfully explain to people when I have a conflict?	
Can I stay quiet when people vent and not offer advice?	
Can I avoid looking for reassurance through social media engagement?	
Can I prevent myself from doing things for other people without being asked?	
Can I engage in leisure activities alone?	

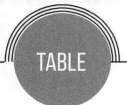
CO-DEPENDENCE VERSUS INTERDEPENDENCE

CO-DEPENDENCE	INTERDEPENDENCE
◊ Possessiveness ◊ People in relationship are guarded	◊ Each individual in the relationship feels freedom and promotion of growth ◊ Each partner is focused on the other's personal development
◊ Threatened by difference ◊ Enmeshed identities ◊ Desire to be just like one another	◊ Partners maintain separate identities ◊ Partners value differences in each other ◊ Both partners are reliant on each other having good self-esteem
◊ Focus of relationship is controlling the other person	◊ Goal of relationship is separate people working toward a mutual goal
◊ Cycles of ups and downs	◊ Able to maintain an attitude of mutual respect and consistency
◊ Desire to crowd out people or activities that don't include both partners	◊ Desire for outside activities for each partner that will bring balance and growth to the relationship
◊ One partner reacts to the mood of the other, taking on their mood state	◊ You can sympathize, but do not take on the partner's problems as your own

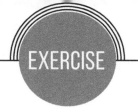
INTERDEPENDENCE INVENTORY

Answer the following questions honestly and thoroughly. Then on the right, mark on a scale of 1 to 5, with 1 being struggling and 5 mastering, how well you've done in the past at this skill, and how well you're doing now.

	PAST	NOW
How well am I supporting my partner's individuality?		
Am I doing activities to improve my self-esteem so that I bring more of myself to the relationship?		
Am I supportive of my partner doing activities to promote a healthy balance?		
Am I able to listen to and sympathize with my partner's challenges without rescuing or worrying to the point of preoccupation?		

Then, whichever has the lowest score *now*, that is what you should work on first.

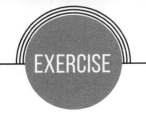

Frequently, patients say to me that they're afraid that saying "no" is going to come across as mean. But it absolutely doesn't have to. Assertive mindful communication is just honest and can be done in a firm and respectful way. Be clear, direct, and if it's in person, make eye contact, and look relaxed. Take ownership of what is 100% within your rights by using "I" statements. Here are some examples:

1. I'd really love to be able to help you, but unfortunately, I'm already committed at that time.

2. What you're going through sounds so hard. I love you and I'm here for you.

3. That activity sounds like a lot of fun. I don't think it's exactly for me, but I'd love to do something else with you at another time.

4. Thank you for offering to include us in your holiday celebration. I really love spending time with family and as much as I'd love to be there, I'm struggling because I remember how much traffic we sat in last year. I'm trying to figure out a compromise.

When people seek to please others in order to feel loved and worthy, their reinforcement for their self-worth comes from outside of themselves. It comes only with the approval given to them from others, but outside reassurance is fickle and unreliable. When it doesn't come, and inevitably it won't, that will only erode our self-confidence. However, self-confidence built from within is not transient; it is the basis for living a life sustainably satisfied, while generating a belief in our lovability.

CHAPTER 7

ACTIVE
SELF-REINFORCEMENT

If you've been doing the exercises in each chapter, I hope you're starting to connect the dots and see how all the components that I've been sharing with you are interrelated. They all involve making better choices for yourself and taking control of your life. I've also tried to demonstrate that getting on the path to achieve Sustainable Life Satisfaction is challenging. Once you begin to experience the positive results, it will become contagious and you'll want to achieve more.

But to achieve more, or simply retain the gains you've made, it's vital to continue these practices long-term. In order to prevent cognitive disintegration of the techniques you've learned, these skills need to be exercised regularly in the same way you would any other muscle in your body.

That's one of the reasons why self-reinforcement is so important. I began learning about self-reinforcement in graduate school while studying anger

IN ORDER TO PREVENT COGNITIVE DISINTEGRATION OF THE TECHNIQUES YOU'VE LEARNED, THESE SKILLS NEED TO BE EXERCISED REGULARLY IN THE SAME WAY YOU WOULD ANY OTHER MUSCLE IN YOUR BODY.

control for my thesis. Self-reinforcement is a powerful tool taught to people looking to control anger. Albert Bandura talked about the importance of having multiple tangible reinforcers at our disposal as rewards. What does that really mean?

Solely rewarding yourself verbally doesn't work to self-reinforce.

But, in order to learn to close, reduce people-pleasing behaviors, make decisions, avoid assumptions and face fears, it is critical to actively self-reinforce.

Why Verbal Reinforcement Doesn't Work

This goes back to Minimizing and Maximizing in Chapter One. I like to tease my clients who Maximize and Minimize. I tell them if they heard a particular compliment one million times it would never be enough. And even if they heard it one million more times, they still wouldn't be satisfied, because they don't believe it. Human beings are not easily fooled by receiving compliments that they think they don't deserve. If they feel undeserving, it just reinforces feelings of inadequacy or imposter syndrome.

You are the best judge of your performance in life. You are the change agent, so you are your best evaluator. But, telling yourself you did a good job is just not enough.

The Power of Tangible Reinforcers

It's critical to have a list of tangible reinforcers. Use them as you are becoming who you want to be. Use them when you feel you've completed the tasks I've suggested. If you faced a fear every day this week, if you closed, if you made a decision, then self-reinforce over the weekend. Reinforcement is key. If you reinforce yourself, you will own your value and lovability in the world.

Whatever it is that you decide to do for yourself, make sure you specifically identify the task as something that you're doing as a reward. Tell yourself you're doing this activity because you are doing a good job working toward achieving your potential.

This sounds easy, but it can be very difficult to do. I give this homework assignment daily to clients. When I check-in the next week, most have not reinforced themselves, even if they made progress toward their goals.

But it's important to recognize that you have the same value as anyone to whom you would give these tangible rewards. You are giving yourself these rewards when *you've* decided you've earned them. If you work for them, then you have to be willing to accept that praise from yourself. Don't delegate reinforcement to others. Learn to own and celebrate your value.

The decreased need for approval from others and the increase in self-reliance to determine the reward for your actions serves to increase self-confidence and decrease feelings of inadequacy.

IT'S IMPORTANT TO RECOGNIZE THAT YOU HAVE THE SAME VALUE AS ANYONE TO WHOM YOU WOULD GIVE THESE TANGIBLE REWARDS.

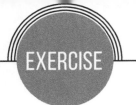

Go through this list and check off the reinforcers that sound enticing to you. Then add to the list your own personal favorite rewards. Set a goal of which SLS challenges you're going to meet this week and which reinforcement you're going to give yourself.

1. Reading a book
2. Listening to music
3. Going dancing
4. Taking a bubble bath
5. Eating a special meal
6. Doing a craft activity
7. Talking to friends
8. Going out
9. Going to a park
10. Going to a movie

11. Getting a massage
12. Buying yourself flowers
13. Going to a sporting event
14. Getting spa services
15. Getting your shoes shined
16. _____
17. _____
18. _____
19. _____
20. _____

This week I am going to _____ at least ____ times. When I do, I am going to reward myself by _____.

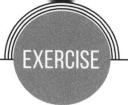
Ask yourself at the end of each day:

What strengths did I show today? _____

_____

What were my challenges? _____

_____

Have I been honest with myself? _____

_____

How did I feel about myself today? _____

_____

What did I close today? _____

_____

What fear did I face today? _____

_____

Did I avoid assumptions today? _____

_____

Was I able to avoid people-pleasing behaviors? _____

_____

What decisions did I make on my own? _____

_____

If I earned reinforcement, did I give it to myself? _____

_____

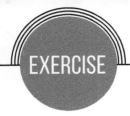

Write your overall goal, say, for example, getting a promotion. Know that your personal goal is outside of your control because it is impacted by the outside world. Then, write what you believe are concrete steps within your control, which will bring you closer to your goal. This could be getting to work early and staying late, completing projects on time, etc. You can pick anything as long as it is not affected by variables in the outside world. It has to be in your control.

Then you have to determine your effectiveness at completing the concrete steps. This evaluation has to be done by you, and not manufactured by reinforcement or reassurance from the outside world. Anything above an 8 is squarely in the Reinforcement Zone. Once you evaluate yourself, reward yourself accordingly.

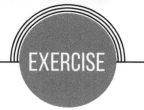

EXERCISE — WEEKLY SELF-EVALUATION

	GOAL	CONCRETE STEP(S):	WEEKLY EVALUATION (1-10)
MONDAY			
TUESDAY			
WEDNESDAY			
THURSDAY			
FRIDAY			
SATURDAY			
SUNDAY			

CONCLUSION

Above all, I want to stress to you that this is a journey and the goal *is* the journey, not perfection. Success is self-acceptance and self-love. Which may mean there are certain skills you don't ever entirely master, you simply increase your self-awareness of them. But if you are able to shift into a mindset of, "I didn't avoid people-pleasing entirely today, but I came close. Which is so much better than before. And I'll come even closer tomorrow. And that's enough. That's worth being proud of myself for," I consider that a huge victory.

Any scales in this workbook are never meant to be used as an excuse to beat yourself up. That would be entirely counter-productive. They are just there as a guidepost, as information to track your progress. And progress is truly what we're after.

START TODAY.

One of the best things about teaching Sustainable Life Satisfaction is the high patient turnover. Nothing gives me greater satisfaction than when someone comes into my office, a few months after we've first met, visibly different than how they arrived. They have a bounce in their step, stand taller, smile more easily, and seem more serene and confident. The way they talk is markedly different, more balanced and content. They are ready to go out on their own.

They have greatly reduced their Thinking Errors, learned to modulate their moods, are consistently incorporating and employing my 6 techniques, and they feel that sense of satisfaction, a core belief in their inherent lovability that has eluded them.

If you do the same, you can have the same. Start today. Right now. If you master all of these strategies in unison, you will attain something so much better than happiness. Something that lasts.

ABOUT THE AUTHOR

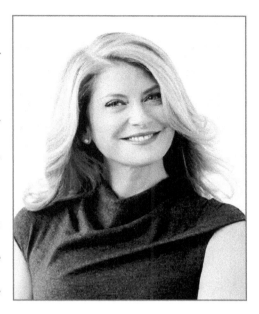

Dr. Jennifer Guttman is a leading clinical psychologist and cognitive behaviorist, with over 20 years of experience in the field of mental health. She has built thriving practices in New York and Connecticut that provide services to over 75 clients a week.

In that time, Jennifer has developed a treatment theory that encompasses some of the fundamental techniques of traditional Cognitive Behavioral Therapy but pushes clients to create a blueprint for self-reliance so they can maintain Sustainable Life Satisfaction^{SM} after treatment.

Presently, 40% of Jennifer's clientele suffer from some serious form of mental illness: bipolar disorder, schizoaffective disorder and major depressive disorder. The other 60% come to see her for transient or developmental life issues. She works with children as young as seven, through individuals in their eighties.

Published in the area of cognitive behavioral therapy and anger control for adolescents, Dr. Guttman has lectured around the country on effective cognitive behavioral techniques for treating mental health issues, and also mentors students in the doctoral program at Long Island University.

Jennifer balances this energizing career with being a mother of two teenagers. And in her little spare time, she fuels her passion for theatre by adding another Playbill to her collection.

CPSIA information can be obtained
at www.ICGtesting.com
Printed in the USA
LVHW061923160123
737227LV00026B/588